SJOGREN SYNDROME JUICING COOKBOOK FOR SENIORS

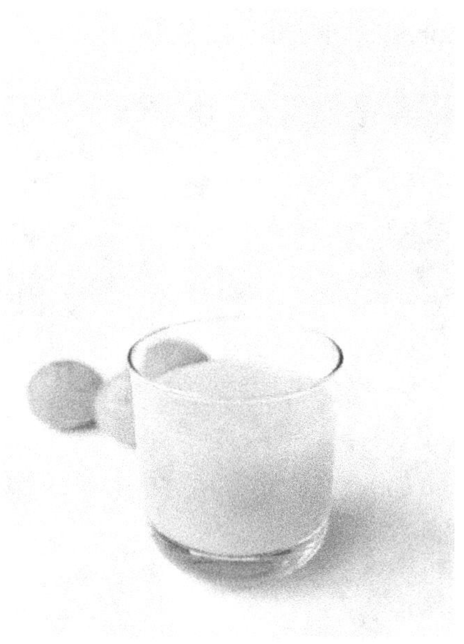

DR. JESSICA SMITH

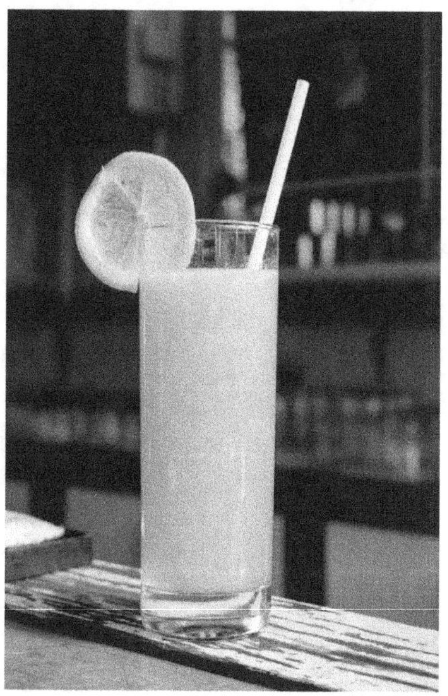

TABLE OF CONTENTS

CHAPTER ONE

How to Use this Cookbook

Understand Your Dietary Needs:

Begin by familiarizing yourself with the dietary needs associated with Sjogren's Syndrome. Recognize the importance of staying hydrated and incorporating anti-inflammatory ingredients.

Consult with a Healthcare Professional:

Before starting any new diet, especially one tailored for specific health conditions like Sjogren's Syndrome, consult with your healthcare professional to ensure the dietary plan aligns with your individual health requirements.

Acquire the Cookbook:

Obtain a copy of the Sjogren Syndrome Juicing Cookbook for Seniors. Look for recipes that emphasize hydrating fruits, vegetables, and ingredients with anti-inflammatory properties.

Gather Ingredients: Collect the ingredients specified in the chosen recipes. Focus on incorporating hydrating fruits like watermelon and cucumber, as well as foods rich in omega-3 fatty acids and antioxidants.

Prepare Your Juicer:

Ensure your juicer is clean and ready for use. Follow the manufacturer's instructions for assembly and operation.

Follow the Recipes:

Stick to the recipes provided in the cookbook. Pay attention to portion sizes and the specific combination of fruits and vegetables suggested for their potential benefits in managing Sjogren's Syndrome symptoms.

Experiment with Flavors:

Feel free to experiment with flavors based on your personal preferences while keeping the recommended ingredients in mind. Adjust sweetness or acidity levels as needed.

Integrate Juicing into Daily Routine:

Make juicing a part of your daily routine. Whether it's a refreshing morning drink or an afternoon pick-me-up, consistency is key to experiencing potential health benefits.

Stay Hydrated: Emphasize hydration throughout the day. Besides juicing, ensure you are consuming an adequate amount of water to combat potential dryness associated with Sjogren's Syndrome.

Monitor How You Feel:

Pay attention to how your body responds to the juicing regimen. Monitor changes in energy levels, hydration, and any improvements in symptoms. If needed, consult your healthcare professional for adjustments.

Understanding Sjogren Syndrome Juicing for Seniors

Understanding Sjogren's Syndrome Juicing for seniors involves recognizing the unique challenges and dietary considerations associated with this autoimmune condition. Sjogren's Syndrome primarily affects the glands responsible for producing moisture, leading to symptoms like dry eyes and mouth.

Incorporating juicing into the diet for seniors with Sjogren's Syndrome aims to address hydration and nutritional needs while considering the potential anti-inflammatory benefits of certain ingredients.

In this context, the Sjogren Syndrome Juicing Cookbook for Seniors becomes a valuable resource.

The recipes are curated to include hydrating fruits and vegetables, such as watermelon, cucumber, and celery, which can assist in combating the dryness commonly experienced by individuals with Sjogren's Syndrome.

Additionally, ingredients rich in omega-3 fatty acids, antioxidants, and vitamins are emphasized to potentially alleviate inflammation and support overall health.

Juicing offers a convenient and palatable way for seniors to consume essential nutrients, especially when dealing with challenges related to chewing or swallowing.

The emphasis on hydration aids in maintaining mucous membranes and supporting bodily functions affected by Sjogren's Syndrome.

However, it's crucial for seniors to consult with healthcare professionals before adopting any new dietary approach.

Tailoring the juicing regimen to individual health needs ensures a personalized and effective strategy for managing Sjogren's Syndrome symptoms and promoting overall well-being in the senior population.

Principles of Sjogren Syndrome Juicing for Seniors

The principles of juicing for seniors with Sjogren's Syndrome revolve around creating nourishing and hydrating beverages that address the unique challenges posed by this autoimmune condition.

These principles aim to mitigate symptoms associated with dryness, inflammation, and potential nutritional deficiencies:

Hydration Focus:

The primary principle is to prioritize hydration. Incorporating fruits and vegetables with high water content, such as watermelon, cucumber, and citrus fruits, helps combat the dryness commonly experienced by individuals with Sjogren's Syndrome.

Anti-Inflammatory Ingredients: Emphasizing ingredients known for their anti-inflammatory properties is crucial. Ingredients like leafy greens, berries, and ginger may contribute to reducing inflammation, potentially alleviating symptoms associated with the syndrome.

Omega-3 Fatty Acids:

Introducing ingredients rich in omega-3 fatty acids, such as flaxseeds or chia seeds, supports overall health and may have anti-inflammatory effects beneficial for individuals with autoimmune conditions.

Vitamin and Antioxidant-Rich Choices:

Selecting fruits and vegetables high in vitamins and antioxidants helps address potential nutritional deficiencies common in individuals with autoimmune disorders.

Balanced Nutrition:

Ensuring a balance of macronutrients and micronutrients is crucial for overall health. Incorporating a variety of fruits, vegetables, and other nutrient-dense ingredients contributes to a well-rounded nutritional profile.

Personalization: Recognizing that individual responses to foods may vary, the juicing approach should be personalized. Seniors should monitor how their bodies respond to specific ingredients and adjust the juicing regimen accordingly.

Consultation with Healthcare Professionals:

The foundational principle is consulting with healthcare professionals before implementing significant dietary changes. Considering individual health conditions and medications ensures that the juicing approach aligns with overall health goals.

Benefits of Sjogren Syndrome Juicing for Seniors

The benefits of juicing for seniors with Sjogren's Syndrome are multifaceted, offering a holistic approach to managing symptoms and promoting overall well-being.

Hydration Support:

Juicing incorporates high-water-content fruits and vegetables, aiding in optimal hydration. This is especially crucial for seniors with Sjogren's Syndrome, who may experience dryness in the eyes and mouth.

Nutrient Absorption: Juicing allows seniors to easily absorb essential nutrients from fruits and vegetables.

This is particularly advantageous for individuals with Sjogren's Syndrome, who may face challenges related to nutrient absorption.

Anti-Inflammatory Properties:

Many juicing ingredients, such as leafy greens, berries, and ginger, possess anti-inflammatory properties. This can help alleviate inflammation associated with Sjogren's Syndrome, contributing to reduced discomfort.

Vitamin and Antioxidant Intake:

Juicing provides a concentrated source of vitamins and antioxidants crucial for immune health. Seniors can benefit from enhanced levels of nutrients to support their immune systems.

Alleviation of Dryness Symptoms:

The hydrating nature of juicing may help mitigate dryness symptoms common in Sjogren's Syndrome, such as dry eyes and mouth, providing relief and improving overall comfort.

Easy Nutritional Access: For seniors who may experience challenges with chewing or swallowing, juicing offers a convenient and palatable way to access essential nutrients without placing additional strain on their digestive system.

Digestive Health:

Juicing may contribute to improved digestive health, aiding seniors who may experience gastrointestinal issues associated with autoimmune conditions.

Customization and Personalization:

The versatility of juicing allows seniors to customize their drinks based on individual preferences and sensitivities, ensuring a personalized approach to nutrition.

Mood and Energy Enhancement:

The abundance of vitamins and minerals in juiced fruits and vegetables can contribute to improved energy levels and may positively impact mood, fostering a sense of vitality.

Holistic Well-Being:

Beyond symptom management, juicing promotes a holistic approach to well-being, empowering seniors to actively participate in their health journey and fostering a positive relationship with nourishment.

Incorporating juicing into the daily routine of seniors with Sjogren's Syndrome can offer a refreshing and nourishing strategy to enhance hydration, nutrient intake, and overall quality of life.

Tips on Sjogren Syndrome Juicing for Seniors

Tips on juicing for Sjogren's Syndrome in seniors involve a thoughtful and tailored approach to address specific symptoms and nutritional needs associated with this autoimmune condition:

Consultation with Healthcare Professionals:

Before initiating any juicing regimen, seniors should consult with their healthcare professionals to ensure that the chosen ingredients align with their individual health conditions, medications, and dietary requirements.

Choose Hydrating Ingredients:

Prioritize hydrating fruits and vegetables, such as watermelon, cucumber, and citrus fruits, to address the dryness symptoms associated with Sjogren's Syndrome.

Include Omega-3 Fatty Acids: Incorporate ingredients rich in omega-3 fatty acids, like flaxseeds or chia seeds, for their potential anti-inflammatory benefits and overall health support.

Experiment with Anti-Inflammatory Herbs:

Explore herbs like turmeric and ginger known for their anti-inflammatory properties, which may help alleviate discomfort associated with inflammation.

Personalize Recipes:

Tailor juicing recipes based on individual preferences and sensitivities. Experiment with ingredient combinations to find flavors that are both enjoyable and supportive of overall health.

Consider Digestive-Friendly Ingredients:

Seniors with digestive concerns should consider ingredients that are gentle on the digestive system, such as mint or aloe vera, to promote digestive health.

Moderation with Sugars: Be mindful of sugar content in fruits and sweeteners. Opt for low-glycemic fruits and limit added sugars to manage blood sugar levels effectively.

Rotate Ingredients:

Introduce variety into juicing recipes by rotating ingredients. This ensures a diverse range of nutrients and minimizes the risk of developing sensitivities to specific foods.

Monitor Hydration Levels:

In addition to juicing, seniors should stay mindful of overall hydration. Incorporate other hydrating beverages and foods to maintain optimal fluid balance.

Listen to Your Body:

Pay attention to how your body responds to different ingredients and adjust the juicing routine accordingly. If any adverse reactions occur, consult with healthcare professionals.

By following these tips, seniors can embark on a juicing journey that not only addresses the symptoms of Sjogren's Syndrome but also contributes to a flavorful and nourishing approach to overall well-being.

Guidelines for juicing with Sjogren's Syndrome in seniors involve a balanced and cautious approach to support symptom management and overall well-being:

Medical Consultation:

Always consult with healthcare professionals before starting a juicing regimen. Individual health conditions, medications, and dietary restrictions need to be considered to ensure a safe and beneficial approach.

Emphasize Hydration:

Prioritize hydrating ingredients to combat the dryness associated with Sjogren's Syndrome. Water-rich fruits like watermelon, cucumber, and berries can contribute to overall hydration.

Include Anti-Inflammatory Elements:

Integrate anti-inflammatory ingredients, such as turmeric, ginger, and leafy greens, to potentially alleviate inflammation associated with Sjogren's Syndrome.

Moderate Sugar Intake:

Seniors should be mindful of sugar content, opting for naturally sweet fruits and minimizing added sugars to manage blood sugar levels effectively.

Diversify Ingredients:

Incorporate a diverse range of fruits, vegetables, and herbs to ensure a variety of nutrients. This promotes overall health and helps avoid potential sensitivities.

Be Mindful of Digestive Sensitivities:

Consider digestive-friendly ingredients, such as mint or aloe vera, to support seniors with potential digestive concerns.

Avoid Overconsumption: While juicing provides concentrated nutrients, it's crucial not to overconsume. Moderation is key to maintaining a balanced diet and preventing excessive caloric intake.

Monitor Blood Sugar Levels:

Seniors with diabetes or blood sugar concerns should monitor their levels closely and choose fruits with lower glycemic indexes.

Adapt Recipes to Preferences: Tailor juicing recipes to individual preferences to ensure an enjoyable experience. Experiment with flavors while adhering to recommended guidelines.

Maintain Overall Hydration:

While juicing is beneficial, seniors should not solely rely on it for hydration. Continue to incorporate other hydrating beverages and foods into the daily routine.

Causes of Sjogren Syndrome

Sjogren's Syndrome is a chronic autoimmune disorder characterized by the immune system mistakenly attacking the body's moisture-producing glands, leading to dryness primarily in the eyes and mouth.

The exact cause of Sjogren's Syndrome remains unclear, but several factors are believed to contribute to its development:

Autoimmune Dysfunction:

The prevailing theory is that an underlying genetic predisposition coupled with environmental triggers may lead to an autoimmune response.

In Sjogren's Syndrome, the immune system attacks healthy tissues, especially the glands responsible for producing saliva and tears.

Genetic Factors:

There appears to be a genetic component, as the condition is more common in individuals with a family history of autoimmune diseases. Specific genetic markers may increase susceptibility to autoimmune responses.

Hormonal Influence:

Hormonal factors, particularly in women, might play a role. The majority of individuals diagnosed with Sjogren's Syndrome are women, and hormonal fluctuations, such as those occurring during menopause, may contribute to symptom onset.

Viral Infections:

Certain viral infections, such as Epstein-Barr virus, have been linked to an increased risk of developing autoimmune disorders, including Sjogren's Syndrome. Viruses may trigger an abnormal immune response.

Environmental Factors:

Exposure to environmental factors, including certain infections or toxins, may contribute to the development of autoimmune diseases. These factors may act as triggers in individuals with a genetic predisposition.

Understanding the causes of Sjogren's Syndrome is a complex and ongoing area of research.

While these factors provide insights into potential triggers, the interplay between genetics, the immune system, and environmental elements is still not fully elucidated.

Research continues to deepen our understanding of the origins of Sjogren's Syndrome, paving the way for improved diagnostic and therapeutic approaches.

Types of Sjogren Syndrome

Sjogren's Syndrome presents in two primary forms: primary Sjogren's Syndrome and secondary Sjogren's Syndrome, each with distinct characteristics:

Primary Sjogren's Syndrome (pSS):

Primary Sjogren's Syndrome occurs when the condition manifests on its own without being associated with another autoimmune disorder. This form predominantly affects the exocrine glands, leading to symptoms such as dry eyes, dry mouth, and potential systemic complications.

Individuals with pSS may experience fatigue, joint pain, and other systemic manifestations beyond glandular involvement.

Secondary Sjogren's Syndrome (sSS):

Secondary Sjogren's Syndrome is diagnosed when an individual has both Sjogren's Syndrome and another autoimmune disorder, typically rheumatoid arthritis or systemic lupus erythematosus.

In sSS, the symptoms and complications of Sjogren's Syndrome may overlap with those of the primary autoimmune condition, leading to a more complex clinical picture.

Both forms of Sjogren's Syndrome share common symptoms, such as dry eyes and dry mouth, but secondary Sjogren's Syndrome tends to present with additional features associated with the accompanying autoimmune disorder.

Diagnosis involves a thorough examination of symptoms, autoimmune markers, and, in some cases, salivary gland biopsies to confirm the presence of characteristic immune cell infiltrates.

Symptoms of Sjogren Syndrome

Sjogren's Syndrome is characterized by a range of symptoms that primarily affect the moisture-producing glands, leading to dryness in various parts of the body. The symptoms can vary in severity and may include:

Dry Eyes:

Persistent dryness, irritation, and a gritty sensation in the eyes are common symptoms. This can lead to blurred vision and an increased sensitivity to light.

Dry Mouth:

Insufficient saliva production causes a dry mouth, making swallowing and speaking challenging. This can contribute to an increased risk of dental issues and oral infections.

Fatigue: Many individuals with Sjogren's Syndrome experience persistent fatigue, which can significantly impact daily activities and overall quality of life.

Joint Pain and Stiffness:

Sjogren's Syndrome can cause joint pain and stiffness, resembling symptoms of rheumatoid arthritis. This can affect multiple joints and lead to decreased mobility.

Swelling and Pain in Salivary Glands:

Inflammation of the salivary glands, particularly those located behind the jaw and in front of the ears, can cause pain and swelling.

Skin and Vaginal Dryness:

Dryness can extend to the skin, leading to irritation and a feeling of tightness. Vaginal dryness may also occur, causing discomfort and pain during sexual activity.

Persistent Cough:

Dryness in the airways may result in a chronic, persistent cough. This can be accompanied by difficulty swallowing.

Cognitive Issues:

Some individuals may experience difficulties with concentration, memory, and cognitive function, often referred to as "brain fog."

Increased Dental Problems:

Decreased saliva production contributes to dental issues such as cavities, gum disease, and an increased risk of oral infections.

Systemic Complications:

In some cases, Sjogren's Syndrome can lead to systemic complications, affecting organs such as the lungs, kidneys, and nervous system.

These symptoms can significantly impact the quality of life for individuals with Sjogren's Syndrome.

Risk Factors of Sjogren Syndrome

The development of Sjogren's Syndrome involves a combination of genetic, hormonal, and environmental factors.

While the exact cause remains elusive, several risk factors contribute to the likelihood of developing this autoimmune condition:

Gender: Sjogren's Syndrome predominantly affects women, with approximately 90% of diagnosed cases occurring in females. The reasons for this gender disparity are not fully understood, but hormonal influences may play a role.

Age:

Although Sjogren's Syndrome can occur at any age, the risk increases with advancing age. The majority of diagnoses occur in individuals over the age of 40, emphasizing age as a significant risk factor.

Genetics:

There is a genetic component to Sjogren's Syndrome, as individuals with a family history of autoimmune disorders, including Sjogren's Syndrome, have an increased risk. Specific genetic markers may contribute to the susceptibility to autoimmune responses.

Autoimmune Diseases:

Individuals with a history of other autoimmune diseases, such as rheumatoid arthritis or systemic lupus erythematosus, are at an elevated risk of developing secondary Sjogren's Syndrome.

Infections:

Certain viral infections, particularly those related to the Epstein-Barr virus, have been associated with an increased risk of Sjogren's Syndrome. Infections may act as triggers for the autoimmune response in genetically predisposed individuals.

Environmental Factors:

Exposure to certain environmental factors, such as toxins or pollutants, may contribute to the development of autoimmune disorders. However, the specific environmental triggers for Sjogren's Syndrome are still under investigation.

Understanding these risk factors provides valuable insights into the complex interplay of genetic and environmental influences that contribute to the onset of Sjogren's Syndrome.

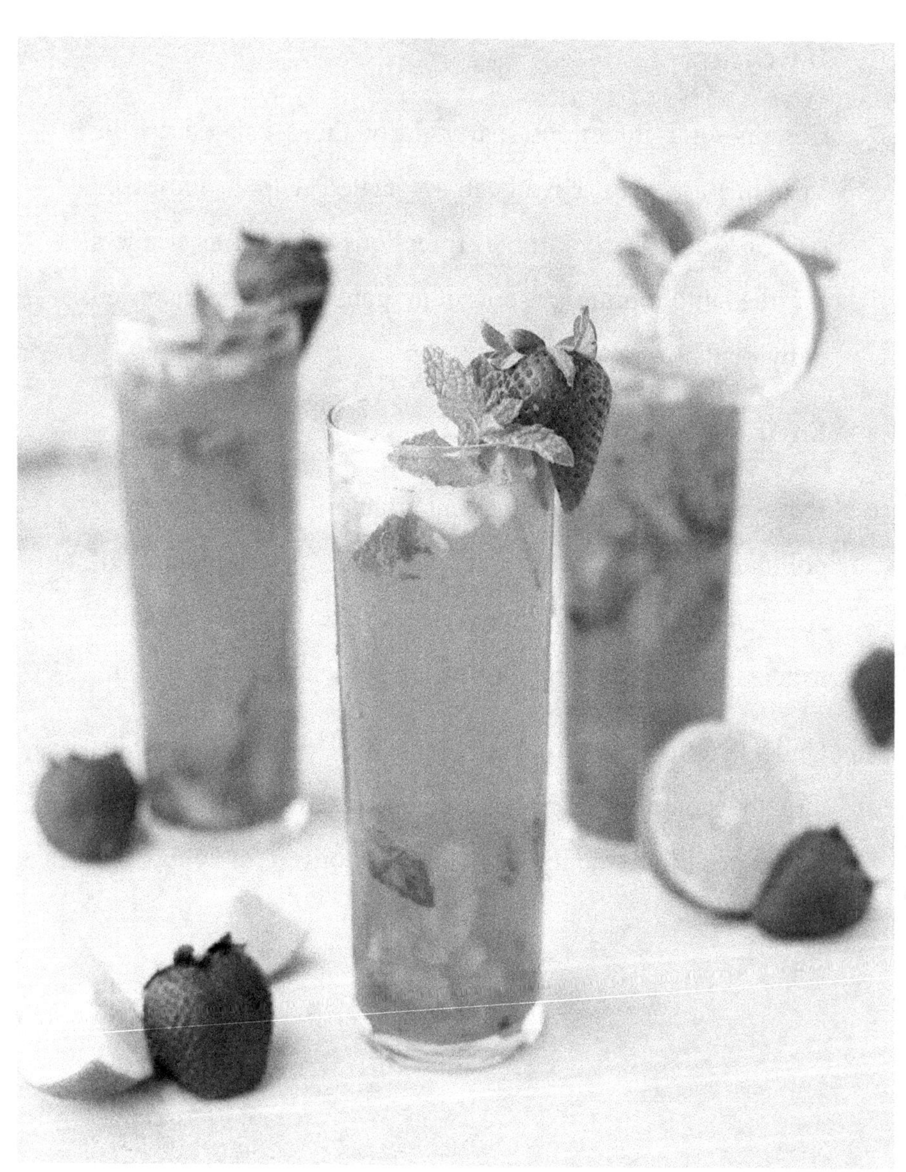

CHAPTER TWO

1: Hydration Boosting Green Citrus Blend

Ingredients:

- 1 cup spinach leaves
- 1 cucumber, peeled and sliced
- 1 green apple, cored and sliced
- 1/2 lemon, peeled
- 1-inch piece of ginger, peeled
- 1 cup coconut water
- Ice cubes (optional)

Instructions:

- Wash and prepare all ingredients.
- In a blender, combine spinach, cucumber, green apple, lemon, and ginger.
- Add coconut water for hydration and blend until smooth.
- Strain the juice if desired for a smoother texture.
- Pour into a glass over ice cubes if preferred.

- Enjoy this refreshing green citrus blend for a hydrating and nutrient-rich boost.

Health Benefits:

- Hydration support from coconut water.
- Anti-inflammatory properties from ginger and spinach.
- Vitamins and antioxidants from green apple and lemon.

Preparation Time: 10 minutes

2: Berry Antioxidant Delight

Ingredients:

- 1 cup mixed berries (blueberries, strawberries, raspberries)
- 1/2 cup Greek yogurt
- 1 tablespoon flaxseeds
- 1 tablespoon honey (optional)
- 1 cup almond milk
- Ice cubes (optional)

Instructions:

- Rinse the berries thoroughly.

- In a blender, combine mixed berries, Greek yogurt, flaxseeds, honey, and almond milk.
- Blend until smooth and creamy.
- Add ice cubes if desired and blend again.
- Pour into a glass and savor the delicious berry antioxidant delight.

Health Benefits:

- Antioxidants from mixed berries.
- Omega-3 fatty acids from flaxseeds.
- Probiotics and protein from Greek yogurt.

Preparation Time: 8 minutes

3: Tropical Immunity Booster

Ingredients:

- 1 cup pineapple chunks
- 1 orange, peeled and segmented
- 1 banana
- 1/2 cup coconut milk
- 1 tablespoon chia seeds
- Ice cubes (optional)

Instructions:

- ➢ Prepare pineapple chunks and orange segments.
- ➢ In a blender, combine pineapple, orange, banana, coconut milk, and chia seeds.
- ➢ Blend until smooth and creamy.
- ➢ Add ice cubes if desired and blend again for a refreshing texture.
- ➢ Pour into a glass and enjoy the tropical flavors of this immunity booster.

Health Benefits:

- ➢ Vitamin C from pineapple and orange for immune support.
- ➢ Electrolytes and hydration from coconut milk.
- ➢ Omega-3 fatty acids from chia seeds.

Preparation Time: 7 minutes

4: Cooling Cucumber Mint Refresher

Ingredients:

- ➢ 1 cucumber, peeled and sliced
- ➢ 1/2 cup fresh mint leaves
- ➢ 1 green apple, cored and sliced

➤ 1 lime, peeled

➤ 1 cup coconut water

➤ Ice cubes (optional)

Instructions:

➤ Prepare cucumber, mint leaves, green apple, and lime.

➤ In a blender, combine cucumber, mint leaves, green apple, lime, and coconut water.

➤ Blend until smooth.

➤ Strain the juice for a smoother consistency.

➤ Pour over ice cubes if desired.

➤ Sip and enjoy the cool and hydrating cucumber mint refresher.

Health Benefits:

➤ Hydration support from cucumber and coconut water.

➤ Digestive aid from mint.

➤ Vitamins and antioxidants from green apple and lime.

Preparation Time: 10 minutes

5: Ginger-Turmeric Anti-Inflammatory Elixir

Ingredients:

- 1-inch ginger, peeled
- 1-inch turmeric, peeled (or 1 teaspoon ground turmeric)
- 1 carrot, peeled and sliced
- 1 orange, peeled and segmented
- 1 cup water
- Honey to taste (optional)

Instructions:

- Prepare ginger, turmeric, carrot, and orange.
- In a blender, combine ginger, turmeric, carrot, orange, and water.
- Blend until smooth.
- Strain if desired for a smoother texture.
- Add honey to taste if sweetness is desired.
- Pour into a glass and indulge in this anti-inflammatory elixir.

Health Benefits:

- ➢ Anti-inflammatory properties from ginger and turmeric.
- ➢ Vitamins and antioxidants from carrot and orange.

Preparation Time: 8 minutes

6: Pineapple-Coconut Hydration Bliss

Ingredients:

- ➢ 1 cup pineapple chunks
- ➢ 1/2 cup cucumber, peeled and sliced
- ➢ 1/2 cup coconut milk
- ➢ 1 tablespoon lime juice
- ➢ 1 tablespoon mint leaves
- ➢ Ice cubes (optional)

Instructions:

- ➢ Prepare pineapple chunks, cucumber, lime juice, and mint leaves.
- ➢ In a blender, combine pineapple, cucumber, coconut milk, lime juice, and mint leaves.
- ➢ Blend until smooth.
- ➢ Add ice cubes if desired and blend again.

➤ Pour into a glass and relish the tropical hydration bliss.

Health Benefits:

➤ Hydration support from pineapple and cucumber.

➤ Electrolytes and healthy fats from coconut milk.

➤ Refreshing flavor with mint and lime.

Preparation Time: 9 minutes

7: Berry Citrus Immune Booster

Ingredients:

➤ 1 cup mixed berries (blueberries, strawberries, raspberries)

➤ 1 orange, peeled and segmented

➤ 1/2 lemon, peeled

➤ 1 tablespoon honey (optional)

➤ 1 cup water

➤ Ice cubes (optional)

Instructions:

➤ Rinse the berries thoroughly.

➤ In a blender, combine mixed berries, orange segments, lemon, honey, and water.

> Blend until smooth.

> Strain if desired for a smoother consistency.

> Add ice cubes if preferred.

> Pour into a glass and enjoy this vitamin-packed immune booster.

Health Benefits:

> Vitamin C and antioxidants from berries, orange, and lemon.

> Natural sweetness with honey (optional).

Preparation Time: 7 minutes

8: Mango-Papaya Tropical Bliss

Ingredients:

> 1 cup mango chunks

> 1/2 cup papaya chunks

> 1 banana

> 1/2 cup coconut water

> 1 tablespoon flaxseeds

> Ice cubes (optional)

Instructions:

> Prepare mango, papaya, banana, and flaxseeds.

- In a blender, combine mango, papaya, banana, coconut water, and flaxseeds.
- Blend until smooth and creamy.
- Add ice cubes if desired and blend again.
- Pour into a glass and savor the tropical flavors of this nutrient-packed bliss.

Health Benefits:

- Vitamin A and C from mango and papaya.
- Omega-3 fatty acids from flaxseeds.
- Hydration support from coconut water.

Preparation Time: 8 minutes

9: Beetroot-Carrot Blood Builder

Ingredients:

- 1 small beetroot, peeled and chopped
- 2 carrots, peeled and sliced
- 1 apple, cored and sliced
- 1/2 lemon, peeled
- 1 cup water
- Honey to taste (optional)

Instructions:

> Prepare beetroot, carrots, apple, and lemon.
> In a blender, combine beetroot, carrots, apple, lemon, and water.
> Blend until smooth.
> Strain for a smoother texture.
> Add honey to taste if sweetness is desired.
> Pour into a glass and enjoy this iron-rich blood-building elixir.

Health Benefits:

> Iron from beetroot for blood health.
> Vitamins and antioxidants from carrots, apple, and lemon.

Preparation Time: 10 minutes

10: Green Tea Infused Citrus Quencher

Ingredients:

> 1 green tea bag, brewed and cooled
> 1 orange, peeled and segmented
> 1/2 lime, peeled
> 1 tablespoon honey

- ➢ 1 cup water

- ➢ Ice cubes (optional)

Instructions:

- ➢ Brew green tea and let it cool.

- ➢ Prepare orange, lime, and honey.

- ➢ In a blender, combine green tea, orange segments, lime, and honey.

- ➢ Blend until well mixed.

- ➢ Strain if desired for a smoother consistency.

- ➢ Add ice cubes if preferred and enjoy this refreshing green tea citrus quencher.

Health Benefits:

- ➢ Antioxidants from green tea.

- ➢ Vitamin C from orange and lime.

- ➢ Natural sweetness with honey.

Preparation Time: 7 minutes

11: Cherry-Almond Antioxidant Blend

Ingredients:

- ➢ 1 cup cherries, pitted

- ➢ 1/2 cup blueberries

- ➢ 1 tablespoon almond butter
- ➢ 1 cup almond milk
- ➢ 1 tablespoon chia seeds
- ➢ Ice cubes (optional)

Instructions:

- ➢ Wash and pit the cherries.
- ➢ In a blender, combine cherries, blueberries, almond butter, almond milk, and chia seeds.
- ➢ Blend until smooth.
- ➢ Add ice cubes if desired and blend again.
- ➢ Pour into a glass and relish the antioxidant-rich cherry-almond blend.

Health Benefits:

- ➢ Antioxidants from cherries and blueberries.
- ➢ Healthy fats and protein from almond butter.
- ➢ Omega-3 fatty acids from chia seeds.

Preparation Time: 9 minutes

12: Avocado-Kale Green Goodness

Ingredients:

- ➢ 1/2 avocado, peeled and pitted

- ➢ 1 cup kale leaves, stems removed
- ➢ 1 green apple, cored and sliced
- ➢ 1/2 lemon, peeled
- ➢ 1 cup coconut water
- ➢ Ice cubes (optional)

Instructions:

- ➢ Prepare avocado, kale, green apple, and lemon.
- ➢ In a blender, combine avocado, kale, green apple, lemon, and coconut water.
- ➢ Blend until creamy and smooth.
- ➢ Add ice cubes if desired and blend again.
- ➢ Pour into a glass and enjoy the nutrient-packed green goodness.

Health Benefits:

- ➢ Healthy fats from avocado.
- ➢ Vitamins and antioxidants from kale, green apple, and lemon.
- ➢ Hydration support from coconut water.

Preparation Time: 8 minutes

13: Pomegranate-Berry Immune Infusion

Ingredients:

- 1/2 cup pomegranate seeds
- 1/2 cup strawberries, hulled
- 1/2 cup blackberries
- 1 tablespoon honey
- 1 cup green tea, brewed and cooled
- Ice cubes (optional)

Instructions:

- Extract pomegranate seeds.
- In a blender, combine pomegranate seeds, strawberries, blackberries, honey, and cooled green tea.
- Blend until well combined.
- Strain for a smoother texture if desired.
- Add ice cubes if preferred and indulge in this immune-boosting infusion.

Health Benefits:

- Antioxidants from pomegranate, strawberries, and blackberries.

> Immune support from green tea.

> Natural sweetness with honey.

Preparation Time: 10 minutes

14: Turmeric-Carrot Anti-Inflammatory Elixir

Ingredients:

> 1 inch turmeric, peeled (or 1 teaspoon ground turmeric)

> 2 carrots, peeled and sliced

> 1 orange, peeled and segmented

> 1 tablespoon fresh ginger, peeled

> 1 cup water

> Honey to taste (optional)

Instructions:

> Prepare turmeric, carrots, orange, and ginger.

> In a blender, combine turmeric, carrots, orange, ginger, and water.

> Blend until smooth.

> Strain for a smoother texture if desired.

> Add honey to taste for sweetness.

- ➢ Pour into a glass and enjoy the anti-inflammatory benefits of this elixir.

Health Benefits:

- ➢ Anti-inflammatory properties from turmeric and ginger.
- ➢ Vitamins and antioxidants from carrots and orange.

Preparation Time: 8 minutes

15: Spinach-Berry Iron Boost

Ingredients:

- ➢ 1 cup spinach leaves
- ➢ 1/2 cup strawberries, hulled
- ➢ 1/2 cup raspberries
- ➢ 1 banana
- ➢ 1 tablespoon hemp seeds
- ➢ 1 cup almond milk
- ➢ Ice cubes (optional)

Instructions:

- ➢ Wash and prepare spinach, strawberries, raspberries, and banana.

> In a blender, combine spinach, strawberries, raspberries, banana, hemp seeds, and almond milk.

> Blend until smooth.

> Add ice cubes if desired and blend again.

> Pour into a glass and relish the iron-boosting goodness.

Health Benefits:

> Iron from spinach for blood health.

> Antioxidants from berries.

> Omega-3 fatty acids from hemp seeds.

Preparation Time: 9 minutes

16: Watermelon-Cucumber Hydration Splash

Ingredients:

> 1 cup watermelon cubes

> 1/2 cucumber, peeled and sliced

> 1 lime, peeled

> 1 tablespoon fresh mint leaves

> 1 cup coconut water

> Ice cubes (optional)

Instructions:

- ➢ Prepare watermelon, cucumber, lime, and mint leaves.
- ➢ In a blender, combine watermelon, cucumber, lime, mint leaves, and coconut water.
- ➢ Blend until smooth.
- ➢ Strain for a smoother consistency if desired.
- ➢ Add ice cubes if preferred and enjoy this hydrating watermelon-cucumber splash.

Health Benefits:

- ➢ Hydration support from watermelon and coconut water.
- ➢ Refreshing flavor with cucumber and mint.
- ➢ Vitamins from lime.

Preparation Time: 7 minutes

17: Blueberry-Almond Protein Power

Ingredients:

- ➢ 1 cup blueberries
- ➢ 1 banana
- ➢ 1 tablespoon almond butter

> 1 cup Greek yogurt

> 1 tablespoon chia seeds

> Ice cubes (optional)

Instructions:

> In a blender, combine blueberries, banana, almond butter, Greek yogurt, and chia seeds.

> Blend until creamy and smooth.

> Add ice cubes if desired and blend again.

> Pour into a glass and enjoy the protein-packed blueberry-almond power.

Health Benefits:

> Protein and probiotics from Greek yogurt.

> Antioxidants from blueberries.

> Healthy fats from almond butter.

Preparation Time: 8 minutes

18: Peach-Basil Relaxation Refresher

Ingredients:

> 1 cup peaches, sliced

> 1/2 cup fresh basil leaves

> 1 pear, cored and sliced

- ➢ 1 tablespoon honey

- ➢ 1 cup chamomile tea, brewed and cooled

- ➢ Ice cubes (optional)

Instructions:

- ➢ Prepare peaches, basil, pear, and brew chamomile tea, letting it cool.

- ➢ In a blender, combine peaches, basil, pear, honey, and chamomile tea.

- ➢ Blend until smooth.

- ➢ Strain for a smoother texture if desired.

- ➢ Add ice cubes if preferred and indulge in the relaxation refresher.

Health Benefits:

- ➢ Relaxing properties from chamomile tea.

- ➢ Vitamins and antioxidants from peaches, pear, and basil.

- ➢ Natural sweetness with honey.

Preparation Time: 9 minutes

19: Pineapple-Mango Joint Soother

Ingredients:

> - 1 cup pineapple chunks
> - 1 cup mango chunks
> - 1 tablespoon turmeric, grated (or 1 teaspoon ground turmeric)
> - 1 cup coconut water
> - 1 tablespoon flaxseeds
> - Ice cubes (optional)

Instructions:

> - Prepare pineapple, mango, turmeric, and flaxseeds.
> - In a blender, combine pineapple, mango, turmeric, coconut water, and flaxseeds.
> - Blend until smooth.
> - Add ice cubes if desired and blend again.
> - Pour into a glass and enjoy the joint-soothing goodness.

Health Benefits:

> - Joint-soothing properties from turmeric.

- ➢ Vitamins and antioxidants from pineapple and mango.
- ➢ Omega-3 fatty acids from flaxseeds.

Preparation Time: 8 minutes

20: Raspberry-Coconut Stress Buster

Ingredients:

- ➢ 1 cup raspberries
- ➢ 1/2 cup coconut milk
- ➢ 1 banana
- ➢ 1 tablespoon honey
- ➢ 1 tablespoon almond butter
- ➢ Ice cubes (optional)

Instructions:

- ➢ In a blender, combine raspberries, coconut milk, banana, honey, and almond butter.
- ➢ Blend until smooth and creamy.
- ➢ Add ice cubes if desired and blend again.
- ➢ Pour into a glass and experience the stress-busting goodness.

Health Benefits:

> ➢ Stress-relieving properties from raspberries.

> ➢ Healthy fats from coconut milk and almond butter.

> ➢ Natural sweetness with honey.

Preparation Time: 7 minutes

21: Kiwi-Strawberry Digestive Bliss

Ingredients:

> ➢ 2 kiwis, peeled and sliced

> ➢ 1 cup strawberries, hulled

> ➢ 1/2 cup Greek yogurt

> ➢ 1 tablespoon chia seeds

> ➢ 1 tablespoon honey

> ➢ 1 cup water

> ➢ Ice cubes (optional)

Instructions:

> ➢ Prepare kiwis and strawberries.

> ➢ In a blender, combine kiwis, strawberries, Greek yogurt, chia seeds, honey, and water.

> ➢ Blend until smooth.

> ➢ Add ice cubes if desired and blend again.

> Pour into a glass and relish the digestive bliss of this kiwi-strawberry concoction.

Health Benefits:

> Digestive support from kiwis and Greek yogurt.
> Antioxidants from strawberries.
> Omega-3 fatty acids from chia seeds.

Preparation Time: 9 minutes

22: Melon-Mint Relaxing Refresher

Ingredients:

> 1 cup honeydew melon, cubed
> 1/2 cup cucumber, peeled and sliced
> 1 tablespoon fresh mint leaves
> 1 tablespoon lime juice
> 1 cup coconut water
> Ice cubes (optional)

Instructions:

> Prepare honeydew melon, cucumber, mint leaves, and lime.
> In a blender, combine honeydew melon, cucumber, mint leaves, lime juice, and coconut water.

- Blend until smooth.
- Strain for a smoother texture if desired.
- Add ice cubes if preferred and enjoy the relaxing refresher.

Health Benefits:

- Hydration support from honeydew melon and coconut water.
- Cooling properties from cucumber and mint.
- Vitamin C from lime.

Preparation Time: 8 minutes

23: Apple-Cranberry Antioxidant Fusion

Ingredients:

- 2 apples, cored and sliced
- 1/2 cup cranberries
- 1 tablespoon fresh ginger, peeled
- 1 cup water
- 1 tablespoon honey
- Ice cubes (optional)

Instructions:

- Prepare apples, cranberries, and ginger.

- ➢ In a blender, combine apples, cranberries, ginger, water, and honey.

- ➢ Blend until smooth.

- ➢ Strain for a smoother consistency if desired.

- ➢ Add ice cubes if preferred and indulge in the antioxidant fusion.

Health Benefits:

- ➢ Antioxidants from apples and cranberries.

- ➢ Digestive aid from ginger.

- ➢ Natural sweetness with honey.

Preparation Time: 10 minutes

24: Mango-Avocado Skin Nourisher

Ingredients:

- ➢ 1 cup mango chunks

- ➢ 1/2 avocado, peeled and pitted

- ➢ 1/2 cup coconut water

- ➢ 1 tablespoon lime juice

- ➢ 1 tablespoon hemp seeds

- ➢ Ice cubes (optional)

Instructions:

> Prepare mango, avocado, lime, and hemp seeds.
> In a blender, combine mango, avocado, coconut water, lime juice, and hemp seeds.
> Blend until creamy and smooth.
> Add ice cubes if desired and blend again.
> Pour into a glass and enjoy the skin-nourishing goodness.

Health Benefits:

> Vitamins and antioxidants from mango and avocado.
> Healthy fats and omega-3 fatty acids from avocado and hemp seeds.
> Hydration support from coconut water.

Preparation Time: 9 minutes

25: Cherry-Pomegranate Joint Elixir

Ingredients:

> 1 cup cherries, pitted
> 1/2 cup pomegranate seeds
> 1 tablespoon flaxseeds
> 1 cup coconut water

> 1 tablespoon honey

> Ice cubes (optional)

Instructions:

> Pit the cherries and extract pomegranate seeds.

> In a blender, combine cherries, pomegranate seeds, flaxseeds, coconut water, and honey.

> Blend until smooth.

> Strain for a smoother texture if desired.

> Add ice cubes if preferred and savor the joint-nourishing elixir.

Health Benefits:

> Anti-inflammatory properties from cherries.

> Antioxidants from pomegranate seeds.

> Omega-3 fatty acids from flaxseeds.

Preparation Time: 8 minutes

26: Spinach-Pineapple Energy Boost

Ingredients:

> 1 cup spinach leaves

> 1 cup pineapple chunks

> 1 banana

➢ 1 tablespoon chia seeds

➢ 1 cup almond milk

➢ Ice cubes (optional)

Instructions:

➢ Wash and prepare spinach leaves.

➢ In a blender, combine spinach, pineapple, banana, chia seeds, and almond milk.

➢ Blend until smooth.

➢ Add ice cubes if desired and blend again.

➢ Pour into a glass and relish the energy-boosting green goodness.

Health Benefits:

➢ Iron from spinach for energy.

➢ Vitamins and antioxidants from pineapple.

➢ Omega-3 fatty acids from chia seeds.

Preparation Time: 9 minutes

27: Raspberry-Coconut Digestive Delight

Ingredients:

➢ 1 cup raspberries

➢ 1/2 cup coconut milk

➤ 1/2 cup Greek yogurt

➤ 1 tablespoon honey

➤ 1 tablespoon flaxseeds

➤ Ice cubes (optional)

Instructions:

➤ In a blender, combine raspberries, coconut milk, Greek yogurt, honey, and flaxseeds.

➤ Blend until creamy and smooth.

➤ Add ice cubes if desired and blend again.

➤ Pour into a glass and enjoy the digestive delight of this raspberry-coconut blend.

Health Benefits:

➤ Probiotics from Greek yogurt for digestive health.

➤ Antioxidants from raspberries.

➤ Healthy fats from coconut milk and flaxseeds.

Preparation Time: 7 minutes

28: Blueberry-Lemon Vitality Infusion

Ingredients:

➤ 1 cup blueberries

➤ 1 lemon, peeled

- ➢ 1 tablespoon fresh ginger, peeled

- ➢ 1 tablespoon honey

- ➢ 1 cup green tea, brewed and cooled

- ➢ Ice cubes (optional)

Instructions:

- ➢ Wash and prepare blueberries, lemon, and ginger.

- ➢ In a blender, combine blueberries, peeled lemon, ginger, honey, and cooled green tea.

- ➢ Blend until well combined.

- ➢ Strain for a smoother texture if desired.

- ➢ Add ice cubes if preferred and savor the vitality infusion.

Health Benefits:

- ➢ Antioxidants from blueberries and green tea.

- ➢ Digestive aid from ginger.

- ➢ Vitamin C from lemon.

Preparation Time: 8 minutes

29: Carrot-Orange Vision Booster

Ingredients:

- ➢ 2 carrots, peeled and sliced
- ➢ 2 oranges, peeled and segmented
- ➢ 1/2 cup Greek yogurt
- ➢ 1 tablespoon flaxseeds
- ➢ 1 tablespoon honey
- ➢ Ice cubes (optional)

Instructions:

- ➢ Prepare carrots, oranges, and honey.
- ➢ In a blender, combine carrots, oranges, Greek yogurt, flaxseeds, and honey.
- ➢ Blend until smooth.
- ➢ Add ice cubes if desired and blend again.
- ➢ Pour into a glass and enjoy the vision-boosting goodness.

Health Benefits:

- ➢ Beta-carotene from carrots for eye health.
- ➢ Vitamin C from oranges.
- ➢ Probiotics from Greek yogurt.

Preparation Time: 9 minutes

30: Pineapple-Cucumber Anti-Inflammatory Cooler

Ingredients:

> 1 cup pineapple chunks
> 1/2 cucumber, peeled and sliced
> 1 tablespoon fresh mint leaves
> 1 tablespoon turmeric, grated (or 1 teaspoon ground turmeric)
> 1 cup coconut water
> Ice cubes (optional)

Instructions:

> Prepare pineapple, cucumber, mint leaves, and turmeric.
> In a blender, combine pineapple, cucumber, mint leaves, turmeric, and coconut water.
> Blend until smooth.
> Strain for a smoother consistency if desired.
> Add ice cubes if preferred and enjoy the anti-inflammatory cooler.

Health Benefits:

> Anti-inflammatory properties from turmeric.

> Hydration support from pineapple and coconut water.

> Cooling effect from cucumber and mint.

Preparation Time: 10 minutes

31: Beetroot-Berry Blood Boost

Ingredients:

> 1 medium-sized beetroot, peeled and sliced

> 1 cup mixed berries (blueberries, raspberries, strawberries)

> 1 tablespoon fresh mint leaves

> 1 tablespoon chia seeds

> 1 cup water

> Ice cubes (optional)

Instructions:

> Prepare beetroot, berries, mint leaves, and chia seeds.

> In a blender, combine beetroot, mixed berries, mint leaves, chia seeds, and water.

> Blend until smooth.

- Strain for a smoother texture if desired.
- Add ice cubes if preferred and enjoy the blood-boosting benefits.

Health Benefits:

- Blood-supporting properties from beetroot.
- Antioxidants from mixed berries.
- Omega-3 fatty acids from chia seeds.

Preparation Time: 8 minutes

32: Mango-Turmeric Immune Elixir

Ingredients:

- 1 cup mango chunks
- 1 tablespoon turmeric, grated (or 1 teaspoon ground turmeric)
- 1/2 lemon, peeled
- 1 tablespoon honey
- 1 cup green tea, brewed and cooled
- Ice cubes (optional)

Instructions:

- Prepare mango, turmeric, lemon, and honey.

- In a blender, combine mango, turmeric, peeled lemon, honey, and cooled green tea.
- Blend until well combined.
- Strain for a smoother texture if desired.
- Add ice cubes if preferred and indulge in the immune-boosting elixir.

Health Benefits:

- Immune support from mango and green tea.
- Anti-inflammatory properties from turmeric.
- Vitamin C from lemon.

Preparation Time: 9 minutes

33: Cabbage-Berry Digestive Detox

Ingredients:

- 1 cup red cabbage, shredded
- 1/2 cup blueberries
- 1/2 cup blackberries
- 1 tablespoon fresh ginger, peeled
- 1 cup water
- 1 tablespoon flaxseeds
- Ice cubes (optional)

Instructions:

> ➢ Prepare red cabbage, blueberries, blackberries, ginger, and flaxseeds.
> ➢ In a blender, combine red cabbage, blueberries, blackberries, ginger, flaxseeds, and water.
> ➢ Blend until smooth.
> ➢ Strain for a smoother texture if desired.
> ➢ Add ice cubes if preferred and enjoy the digestive detox.

Health Benefits:

> ➢ Digestive support from red cabbage and flaxseeds.
> ➢ Antioxidants from berries.
> ➢ Anti-inflammatory properties from ginger.

Preparation Time: 10 minutes

34: Spinach-Pear Iron Infusion

Ingredients:

> ➢ 1 cup spinach leaves
> ➢ 2 pears, cored and sliced
> ➢ 1 tablespoon hemp seeds
> ➢ 1 tablespoon honey

> 1 cup almond milk

> Ice cubes (optional)

Instructions:

> Wash and prepare spinach leaves and pears.

> In a blender, combine spinach, pears, hemp seeds, honey, and almond milk.

> Blend until smooth.

> Add ice cubes if desired and blend again.

> Pour into a glass and enjoy the iron-infusing goodness.

Health Benefits:

> Iron from spinach for blood health.

> Fiber and natural sweetness from pears.

> Omega-3 fatty acids from hemp seeds.

Preparation Time: 9 minutes

35: Pineapple-Kale Skin Revitalizer

Ingredients:

> 1 cup pineapple chunks

> 1 cup kale leaves, stems removed

> 1 cucumber, peeled and sliced

- ➤ 1 tablespoon fresh mint leaves
- ➤ 1 cup coconut water
- ➤ Ice cubes (optional)

Instructions:

- ➤ Prepare pineapple, kale, cucumber, and mint leaves.
- ➤ In a blender, combine pineapple, kale, cucumber, mint leaves, and coconut water.
- ➤ Blend until smooth.
- ➤ Strain for a smoother consistency if desired.
- ➤ Add ice cubes if preferred and enjoy the skin-revitalizing concoction.

Health Benefits:

- ➤ Hydration support from pineapple and coconut water.
- ➤ Skin-nourishing properties from kale and cucumber.
- ➤ Cooling effect from mint.

Preparation Time: 8 minutes

36: Aloe Vera-Berry Gut Soother

Ingredients:

- ➤ 1/4 cup aloe vera gel

> 1 cup mixed berries (strawberries, blueberries, raspberries)
> 1/2 cup Greek yogurt
> 1 tablespoon honey
> 1 cup coconut water
> Ice cubes (optional)

Instructions:

> Extract aloe vera gel from the plant (be sure to remove the yellow latex).
> In a blender, combine aloe vera gel, mixed berries, Greek yogurt, honey, and coconut water.
> Blend until smooth.
> Add ice cubes if desired and blend again.
> Pour into a glass and enjoy the gut-soothing benefits.

Health Benefits:

> Gut-soothing properties from aloe vera.
> Probiotics from Greek yogurt.
> Antioxidants from mixed berries.

Preparation Time: 9 minutes

37: Watermelon-Mint Electrolyte Refresher

Ingredients:

> ➢ 2 cups watermelon cubes
> ➢ 1 tablespoon fresh mint leaves
> ➢ 1 tablespoon chia seeds
> ➢ 1 tablespoon lime juice
> ➢ 1 cup coconut water
> ➢ Ice cubes (optional)

Instructions:

> ➢ Prepare watermelon, mint leaves, chia seeds, and lime.
> ➢ In a blender, combine watermelon, mint leaves, chia seeds, lime juice, and coconut water.
> ➢ Blend until smooth.
> ➢ Strain for a smoother consistency if desired.
> ➢ Add ice cubes if preferred and relish the electrolyte-refreshing goodness.

Health Benefits:

> ➢ Hydration support from watermelon and coconut water.

- Electrolytes from chia seeds.
- Refreshing flavor with mint and lime.

Preparation Time: 8 minutes

38: Avocado-Cucumber Skin Hydrator

Ingredients:

- 1/2 avocado, peeled and pitted
- 1/2 cucumber, peeled and sliced
- 1 tablespoon fresh basil leaves
- 1 tablespoon lime juice
- 1 cup coconut water
- Ice cubes (optional)

Instructions:

- Prepare avocado, cucumber, basil leaves, lime, and coconut water.
- In a blender, combine avocado, cucumber, basil leaves, lime juice, and coconut water.
- Blend until creamy and smooth.
- Add ice cubes if desired and blend again.
- Pour into a glass and enjoy the skin-hydrating concoction.

Health Benefits:

> Healthy fats and vitamins from avocado.

> Hydration support from cucumber and coconut water.

> Antioxidants from basil leaves.

Preparation Time: 7 minutes

39: Cherry-Almond Sleep Inducer

Ingredients:

> 1 cup cherries, pitted

> 1 banana

> 1 tablespoon almond butter

> 1 cup almond milk

> 1 tablespoon honey

> Ice cubes (optional)

Instructions:

> Pit the cherries.

> In a blender, combine cherries, banana, almond butter, almond milk, and honey.

> Blend until smooth.

> Add ice cubes if desired and blend again.

➢ Pour into a glass and enjoy the sleep-inducing blend.

Health Benefits:

➢ Melatonin in cherries promotes better sleep.

➢ Healthy fats from almond butter.

➢ Natural sweetness with honey.

Preparation Time: 9 minutes

40: Peach-Basil Digestive Calmer

Ingredients:

➢ 2 peaches, sliced

➢ 1/4 cup fresh basil leaves

➢ 1 tablespoon fresh ginger, peeled

➢ 1 cup coconut water

➢ 1 tablespoon honey

➢ Ice cubes (optional)

Instructions:

➢ Prepare peaches, basil leaves, ginger, and coconut water.

➢ In a blender, combine peaches, basil leaves, ginger, coconut water, and honey.

➢ Blend until smooth.

➤ Strain for a smoother texture if desired.

➤ Add ice cubes if preferred and enjoy the digestive-calming concoction.

Health Benefits:

➤ Digestive aid from ginger and basil leaves.

➤ Hydration support from peaches and coconut water.

➤ Natural sweetness with honey.

Preparation Time: 8 minutes

CONCLUSION

Embracing a Sjogren Syndrome Juicing lifestyle for seniors isn't just about crafting delicious and refreshing beverages; it's about promoting holistic well-being.

These carefully curated recipes aim to offer not only a symphony of flavors but a harmonious blend of nutrients that may support those managing Sjogren's Syndrome.

Through the infusion of nature's bounty, we strive to address specific health considerations, providing a source of hydration, essential vitamins, and potential anti-inflammatory properties.

Each recipe is a testament to the power of whole, natural ingredients, offering seniors a delightful way to enhance their nutritional intake.

As you embark on this juicing journey, remember that individual responses may vary.

May these Sjogren Syndrome juicing recipes for seniors not only tantalize the taste buds but also contribute to a nourished body, a rejuvenated spirit, and a more vibrant life. Cheers to embracing wellness, one refreshing sip at a time!